KETOGENIC DIET FOR BEGINNERS

Easy Guide to a High-Fat Diet, Low carb, Weight-loss, Regain Energy

Julia Cooper

Table of Contents

INTRODUCTION

Are you struggling with weight loss? Do you want to look leaner, more attractive and filled with energy? Do you want a proven way to lose weight? Then this Ketogenic Diet for Beginners book is for you. No Ketogenic Diet meal plan can ever be successful unless you have a proper information for your diet. In this guide, you'll get all the essentials you will need to lose weight.

The ketogenic diet is not some new fad. It has been studied and developed by health experts since the 1920's. Millions of people have already tried out the Ketogenic Diet and have seen numerous benefits in both their health and energy levels. The book provides a step-by-step strategy that will help you get started and help you make sure you are taking the right steps to lose weight the healthy way.

This Ketogenic Diet For Beginners is both for those starting out the diet and Keto veterans. The tips, tricks, and strategies described in this book are insightful, proven, effective and actionable. With this beginner's book, you have a guide that can be used, not only for education purposes, but as practical advice for action. If you are serious about both losing weight and getting healthier, you need this book. So what are you waiting for? Get your copy today and get started on your weight loss journey. The book is an informative guide on the Ketogenic diet and also contains breakfast, lunch and dinner keto diet recipes.

1

CHAPTER 1

What Is the Keto Diet and Ketosis?

Understanding the Keto Diet

The ketogenic diet, also known as Keto diet, comprises of foods low in carbohydrates, high in fat and moderate in protein to help you maintain a healthy body. Fats make up a big portion of the calories in a Keto diet while proteins and carbohydrates incorporated in smaller amounts. This diet structure encourages your body to rely on your stored fat rather than glucose or blood sugar from carbohydrates for energy. This makeup prevents weight gain and promotes overall improvements in health. The focus of the Keto diet is to limit carbohydrates, infuse enough protein to meet your daily needs and incorporate higher amounts of fat into your diet to meet your energy needs.

What is Ketosis?

The human body has several metabolic pathways to convert the food you eat into energy for daily activity. For the human body, using the glucose from carb-rich food is the default metabolic pathway because glucose is fast acting and easily accessible. However, when you limit your carb consumption, your body turns to fat for energy.

Ketosis

Your body's second favorite source of energy is fat. With Keto, your carb consumption is less, and your body turns to fat to get energy. When this occurs, your liver breaks down fat into fatty acids, then breaks down these fatty acids into an energy-rich element known as ketones or ketone bodies. The existence of Ketone bodies in the blood is known as Ketosis. The goal of the Ketogenic diet is to lift your body into permanent ketosis and to make your body a fat burning machine.

Ketosis and Weight Loss

You know now how the ketones are formed and might be wondering how this helps you to lose weight. When you follow a standard American diet, you eat mostly carb-rich foods; your body burns them for energy and stores any excess as glycogen in your liver and triglycerides in your fat cells. When you limit carbohydrates, your body drains its glycogen storage in the muscles and liver and begins to burn body fat for energy. So when your body starts to burn fat, your fat cells shrink and you start to lose weight and become leaner.

How you Force your Body into Ketosis

Forcing your body into ketosis is not easy, but once you get used to it, it will become easier. The first thing you should do to induce ketosis is to limit your carb consumption. Also, you have to limit your protein consumption as well because your body can convert excess protein into glucose, so it will not need to use fat as fuel. You can induce ketosis by eating a high-fat diet that includes moderate protein and small amount carbohydrate. This is called the ketogenic diet.

- **5–10 percent of calories from carbohydrates**

- **15–30 percent of calories from protein**
- **60–75 percent of calories from fat**

You don't have to worry about calories because fats and proteins will keep you full for a long period. But if you are being strict with your diet, intake to take off excess weight counting can be done.

Fat - 1 gram = 9 calories
Protein - 1 gram = 4 calories
Carbohydrates - 1 gram = 4 calories

You can set calories on the ketogenic percentage ratio and in daily keto food list will be equals: about 70% of calories from fat, about 20% from protein, and under 10% from carbohydrate.

Here's an example on how to do it:

Let's say you set your total calorie intake for the day to be 1500.

(The number of calories you need depends on your age, gender, weight, height, and activity level. If you need to know please use a calorie calculator; Google "calorie calculator")

- 1500 x .70 = 1050 calories from fat = 1050/9 = 116,6 grams of fat
- 1500 x .20 = 300 calories from protein = 300/4 = 75 grams of protein
- 1500 x .10 = 150 calories from carbohydrates = 150/4 = 37,5 grams of carb.

Most people who have experienced ketosis achieved all the great fat loss and health benefits at 20-30 grams of net carbs (or up to 50 grams of total carbs) per day.

Benefits of the Ketogenic Diet

The diet offers many health benefits, including:

- Lower your cravings for food: This is one of the initial benefits of the diet. Fat has a very satisfying and filling presence, and the existence of ketone in your body will naturally lower your appetite. Various studies show that the diet leads to an automatic reduction in appetite.
- Lowers blood pressure: After starting the diet, your blood pressure will stabilize within a few weeks. Various clinical studies show that that the diet leads to a reduced risk of high blood pressure.
- Lower your risk of heart disease: Triglycerides are fat molecules, and excess triglycerides in your blood lead to heart disease. Several studies prove that the diet dramatically lowers blood triglycerides.
- Lower cholesterol: Various studies show that a diet such as Keto helps you lower bad cholesterol and boost good cholesterol levels.
- Boost energy: Following the diet help you to increase your energy levels. If you are suffering from chronic fatigue symptoms, the diet will lower the symptoms.
- Lift your mood: The existence of ketone in your body boosts the production of feel-good hormones such as dopamine and serotonin in your body.
- Reverse type 2 diabetes: Various studies show that Keto diet lowers your blood sugar and insulin levels and helps reverse type 2 diabetes.
- Weight loss: The Keto diet will help you to lower your weight. Various studies show that the diet causes quick weight loss within the first two weeks. The diet is very effective reducing the harmful belly fat.

Who should not follow the Keto Diet?

Some precautions must be made clear:

- Before starting the Keto diet, it is highly recommended that you undergo a health checkup to rule out any medical conditions that interfere with your diet plan.
- Diet is not recommended for people with problems kidney, pancreatic, or pre-existing liver conditions.
- If you have type 1 diabetes or hypoglycemia, then this diet is not for you.
- This diet is not safe for people who have gestational diabetes or are nursing or pregnant.
- The diet is not appropriate for people recovering or suffering from an eating disorder.

The diet is not recommended for the following:

- People with a history of mental health problems
- People who have a fever or feel unwell
- People with a significant medical condition should discuss with their doctor before starting the diet
- People recovering from surgery
- Pregnant women or breastfeeding mothers
- People with type 1 diabetics
- Children under 18 years old
- People who are underweight

The side effects of the Keto diet

Starting the diet can cause a few side effects, including

- Induction Flu: irritability, brain fog, confusion, nausea, lethargy, headache. These symptoms are very common during the first week of the diet.

    The cure: Water and salt: You can minimize or even

completely cure these problems by getting enough salt and water into your system. In a large glass of water, add ½ tsp. salt and drink to reduce or eliminate the symptoms. Repeat once daily. A better option is drinking broth made with bone, beef or chicken.

- Leg Cramps: Leg cramps are a minor issue, but they can be painful.

The cure: Drink plenty of fluids and get enough salt. Also, you can supplement with magnesium. Take 3 slow release magnesium tablets daily for 20 days.

- Constipation: Constipation is another side effect of the diet.

The cure: Get enough salt and drink plenty of fluids. Focus on eating more vegetables or include another source of fiber. Milk of Magnesia can help you prevent constipation.

- Bad breath: Bad breath during a diet is another unpleasant problem.

The Cure

- Maintain a good oral hygiene
- Use a breath freshener regularly
- Get enough salt and drink enough fluid
- Eat a bit more carbs.
- Heart palpitations.

The cure: Getting enough salt and enough fluid is the quickest solution.

All the problems can be cured by increasing your carb consumption.

CHAPTER 2

What to Eat and What to Avoid

In this chapter, we are going to discuss what you can eat and what you have to avoid while on a Ketogenic diet.

What to Eat on a Ketogenic Diet

You can eat from the following food groups:

- Fats and Oils: Get your fats from various meats and nuts. Also include monounsaturated and saturated fats from sources like coconut oil, butter, and olive oil.
- Protein: Focus on eating grass-fed, pasture-raised, organic meat. Eat meat in moderation.
- Vegetables: Eat vegetables that grow above ground, mainly leafy green vegetables.
- Dairy: Buy full-fat dairy products.
- Nuts and seeds: Eat fat-rich nuts such as macadamia and almonds.
- Beverages: Focus on drinking mostly water and broth. Flavor your water with lime/lemon juice and stevia-based flavorings.

Let's discuss the details

Fats and oils

- You can cook with saturated fats: butter, ghee, lard and coconut oil.
- Use monounsaturated fats on salad dressings: olive, avocado, and macadamia nut oil.
- Take polyunsaturated fats: Eat fatty fish and get fat from animal protein. Avoid processed fats such as margarine spread.
- Trans fats: Avoid completely.

Protein

More protein containing: pork chops, ribeye steak, chicken breast, fatty fish, shellfish, ground beef, ground lamb, liver. Less protein containing: eggs, chicken thigh, and bacon.

- Fish: Eat Wild-Caught fish like tuna, cod, halibut, trout, snapper, salmon, mackerel, and catfish. Fattier fish is better.
- Shellfish: Mussels, scallops, crab, lobster, oysters, clams and squid.
- Whole eggs: Try to get free-range.
- Beef: Stew meat, roasts, steak, and ground beef. Choose fattier cuts.
- Pork: Ham, tenderloin, pork chops, pork loin, and ground pork. Avoid meats that include added sugars.
- Poultry: Chicken, pheasant, quail, duck and wild game.
- Offal/Organ: Tongue, kidney, liver, and heart.
- Other meat: Turkey, lamb, goat, veal and other wild game.
- Bacon and Sausage: Avoid anything with added sugar.
- Nut Butter: Focus on natural, unsweetened nuts. Buy fattier version like macadamia and almond nut butter.

Vegetables and Fruit

Eat mostly vegetables that are low in carbs and high in nutrients. Focus on cruciferous vegetables that are leafy, green and grown above ground, like green beans and green bell peppers. Blackberries, raspberries, yellow onion, broccoli, cauliflower, cabbage will give you more carbs and spinach, mushrooms, green bell peppers, green beans, romaine lettuce will give you less carbs.

Limit your intake of:

- Root Vegetables: This includes squash, mushrooms, garlic, parsnip, and onion.
- Nightshades: This includes peppers, eggplants, and tomatoes.
- Citrus: This includes orange, lemon and lime.
- Berries: This includes blueberries, blackberries, and raspberries.
- Completely avoid large fruits like bananas, potatoes, and starchy vegetables.

Dairy Products

Brie, mayonnaise, mozzarella cheese, heavy cream gives you less carbohydrates, and cream cheese, Greek yogurt and cottage cheese, parmesan cheese gives you more carbohydrates.

Dairy you can eat on Keto are:

- Hard cheese, including Parmesan, aged cheddar, Swiss, feta, etc.
- Soft cheese, including monetary jack, Colby, Brie, blue, mozzarella, etc.
- Spreadable including crème Fraiche, mascarpone, sour cream, cream cheese, cottage cheese, etc.

- Mayonnaise
- Heavy whipping cream
- Greek yogurt

Nuts and Seeds

- Fatty, low carb nuts, including pecans, Brazil nuts, and macadamia nuts.
- Fatty, moderate carb nuts, including peanuts, hazelnuts, almonds, walnuts and pine nuts.
- Higher carb nuts, including cashews and pistachios. Eat them occasionally.

Water and Beverages

Commonly consumed beverages on Keto are:

- Water: Drink plenty of water. You can drink sparkling or still water.
- Broth: Broth will help you prevent Keto flu. They are loaded with nutrients and vitamins.
- Coffee: Help you to lose weight and improves mental focus.
- Tea: Try to stick with green or black.
- Coconut and almond milk: Use unsweetened versions.
- Diet Soda: Severely reduce or completely avoid.
- Flavoring: Small packets of stevia or sucralose are fine. Focus on natural flavorings such as a squeeze of lemon or lime in your water.
- Alcohol: Most beer and wine are loaded with the carb. Choose hard liquor.

Spices

You can cook with cinnamon, cumin and cayenne chili powder.

Sprinkle with parsley, cilantro and basil.

Marinate with thyme, rosemary and garlic powder.

Condiments and Sauces

Keto friendly condiments and sauces include:

- Low or no sugar added ketchup
- Hot sauce
- Mustard
- Low or no sugar added sauerkraut
- Cage-free and avocado oil based mayonnaise
- Low or no sugar added relish
- Worcestershire sauce
- Horseradish
- Salad dressings (fattier dressings like Caesar and ranch and unsweetened vinaigrettes)
- Acceptable sweetener added flavored syrups

Try to avoid pre-made condiments.

Sweeteners

Keto recommended sweeteners:

- Stevia: Stevia is highly recommended. Choose the liquid form.
- Sucralose: Many people confuse it with Splenda, but sucralose is different because it is a pure sweetener. Choose liquid version.
- Erythritol: Erythritol is a great choice as a sweetener.
- Monk fruit: This is an uncommon sweetener and used mixed with others.
- Different brands: There are various Keto friendly sweetener brands available in the market.

Hidden Carbs

As a beginner, starting the Keto diet can be a bit difficult for you. Here is a list of common items that have hidden carbs:

- Low-carb products: Avoid any type of low-carb packaged food products, but if you must then read the food labels carefully.
- Spices: Spices contain carbs, and some have more carbs than others. Always read the labels to make sure there is no added sugar in your spice blends.
- Fruit and berries: Due to high sugar content, most fruits are not allowed on Keto.
- Tomato-based products: Tomato-based products are very popular. Before buying read the labels carefully.
- Condiments: Read the labels before buying condiments and sauces.
- Peppers and chiles: Limit small peppers because they are very sweet and a tiny chili paper can contain 3 to 4 grams of carb.
- Diet soda: You can drink diet soda occasionally, but it is recommended that you avoid it completely.
- Chocolate: You can eat chocolate on Keto, but be careful about serving size.
- Medicine: Flu remedies, cough syrups, and cold medications often contain lots of sugar.

Foods to Avoid

Avoid these:

- Grains: Any wheat products (cakes, cereals, pasta, bread, buns), rice, corn, and beer should be avoided. Grains include whole grains like quinoa, buckwheat, barley, rye, and wheat.

- Starch: Avoid vegetables like yams, potatoes and other things like muesli, oats, etc.
- Sugar: Usually found in ice cream, chocolate, candy, sports drinks, juice, and soda. Anything processed and packaged is likely to contain sugar.
- Trans Fats: Avoid anything that contains hydrogenated fats.
- Fruit: Avoid large fruits (bananas, oranges and apples).
- Low-fat foods: Low-fat foods are usually high in sugar and carb.

Online Help to Keep You Interested on the Keto diet.

Keeping track of what you are eating is extremely important when following the ketogenic diet. The Ketogenic diet won't work for you without an accurate record. There is plenty of online help available for you. So just research and find what you need.

For example, Google "Keto Calculator" and you will get a few keto calculator websites.

If you need Keto friendly baking companies, then Google "Keto friendly baking".

Also, if you need calorie calculator, then Google "calorie calculator".

Just Google what you want to know.

Eating Out

When eating in a restaurant, choose to eat only meat, such as steaks without sauce or starchy gravy. Eat meat, egg or green based salads with mayonnaise or oil dressing. Avoid ketchup and use mustard. Here is a guideline how you can order meals according to your keto need:

- Chinese: Eat crispy duck, fish soups, and seafood without noodles. Any meat or egg-based meal is ok. Avoid sweet sauce and starchy vegetables.
- Italian: Order non-starchy vegetables such (fresh, grilled, fried or steamed), seafood and meat-based foods. Avoid starchy sauces and bread crumbs in salads. Ask for balsamic vinegar, olive oil or mayonnaise dressing.
- Greek: Greek cuisine is keto friendly. The cuisine offers you a variety of fish and meat-based dishes. Avoid fries, pita bread, and sweets.
- German: German cuisine is carb based. Choose meat-based dishes such as tartar steak, sauerkraut, and sausages. Avoid meals with bread.
- Indian: Eat meat-based foods, such as tikka dish, curry, korma, and vegetables. Avoid dahl, lentils, vindaloo, rice, potatoes, and naan bread.
- Mexican: Avoid tortillas and beans. Eat meat-based meals and salads.
- Japanese: Avoid rice and eat seafood.
- Turkish: Avoid bread and sugar added foods. Eat vegetables and kebabs.
- Vietnamese: Avoid sugary sauces and noodles. Eat meat-based meals.

For takeaway, choose foods such as kebabs and sushi.

CHAPTER 3

Tips to Make the Diet Work for You

Tips for beginners who want to follow the Ketogenic diet plan

- One of the aims of the Keto diet is to limit your intake of carb-rich foods. Aim for eating 20g per day. Measuring your carb intake is easy so don't worry about consuming too much carb.
- A ketogenic diet contains 60 to 75% fat, 15 to 30% protein and 5 to 10% carbohydrates. The internet is a great help for you to calculate and measure your meals.
- With the ketogenic or keto diet, you are eating less carbs, but careful about eating too much protein. Surplus protein can cause higher levels of insulin production.
- You have to strictly follow the ketogenic diet and can't break the routine even for a day. If you break the routine, then you have to start from the beginning.
- If you are not certain about any food or food item; check and check again before eating it.
- Avoid root vegetables because they are loaded with the carbs.
- For the first month of your diet plan, drink a cup of broth daily. Drinking broth will help to maintain your

body's electrolyte balance, and you will avoid the keto flu.

- Take a few photos of your body from all angles before starting the diet. Compare them after one month. The difference in body fat, especially in the abdomen region will encourage you to stay with the diet plan.
- Read articles, blogs, and columns about the keto diet in the newspapers and on the internet. Also, read books like this and watch videos to know as much as possible.

Tips that will help you to follow the ketogenic diet for life

Often a diet plan requires that the dieter avoids the foods that he or she enjoys eating. This feeling of deprivation is one of the main reasons why diet plans fail. But with the ketogenic diet plan, you only have to avoid carb based foods. So the diet becomes easier to follow. Here are some tips for you:

- Find a caring person who is prepared to give you mental support. The ideal person might be a family member or a friend. Having a compassionate person to support you during the difficult period of diet will help you immensely.
- Consult with your doctor if you think you need additional multi-vitamins and supplements.
- Cook a variety of keto recipes every week. This approach of eating will give you the opportunity to taste different foods. The diet will be unpredictable and exciting, and this will make it easier to maintain the diet.
- Experiment with the ingredients and create your own keto recipes, include food items you enjoy eating. Experimenting and playing around with recipes will

keep you interested in the keto diet.

- Drink lots of water. Water will help you to control craving for foods that are not included in the keto diet. Water will also help remove toxins from your body.
- Develop a schedule for sleep and ensure you are getting enough sleep every night. Studies have shown that people tend to eat more when they are tired or sleep deprived. When you are sleep deprived, your body produces a hormone that forces you to eat more.
- Eat fruits and vegetables as snacks instead of cookies and cupcake. If you feel you are hungry between meals, eat some fruits, seeds, and nuts. They are nutritious and help maintain the diet.
- Eat 5 to 6 times daily and ensure you are not too hungry any time of the day because if you are starving, you will immediately go for carb-rich foods.

Tips for Women

Keto for women is little different. So here are some tips that are particularly important for women during their period:

- Meats take more time to digest. So eat more sugar-free jello, vegetables, and broth while you are having your period.
- Take omega-3: Take omega-3 essential oils from fatty fish such as wild salmon, sardines, organic beef, leafy green, flaxseeds.
- Eat yogurt. While you are following keto, eat low carb yogurt such as "diabetic friendly" yogurt. Yogurt contains "Lactobacillus acidophilus," which is important for vaginal health.
- Drink Vega (whole food shake, no gluten, no soy, or artificial sugar) with almond milk to help balance your

hormones.

- Exercise for your boobs. Weight loss can result in saggy boobs. So do a few pushups daily to keep everything tight up there.
- Keep your pH in check. Drink lemon water every day to keep your pH in check.
- Eat low-carb chocolates. Often during your periods, you have sweet cravings. So eat a handful of low-carb, real dark chocolate.
- Take cranberry supplements. You need cranberry supplements daily to avoid urinary tract infections.

If losing weight is still difficult for you...

Some dieters still find it difficult to lose weight. Here are a few tips for them:

- Check if you are eating an excessive amount of protein. Excessive protein converts into glycogen and stops your body getting into ketosis.
- Avoid taking any artificial sweeteners. Mints, chewing gums, and cough syrup contain sugar and artificial sugars.
- Carb cheating is another reason for weight gain. Avoid carb-rich snacks.
- You may be eating excessive carb-rich foods. So check and lower your carb intake and include coconut oil in your keto diet. Coconut oil contains MCTs, which help your body to enter ketosis.

Even if the dieter's body is in ketosis stage, the following can cause people to find it hard to lose weight.

- A short period of sleep or chronic sleep problem can affect your weight loss goals. The maximum fat loss is achieved with a keto diet, daily exercise, and enough sleep.

- Stress is one of the major factors when it comes to weight loss. Your body produces stress hormone cortisol when you are stressed. This hormone makes losing weight difficult.
- Leptin hormone can prevent weight loss. Leptin signals your brain when to stop eating. With the gradual fat loss, your brain will get fewer signals from leptin. Eat food rich in fat and protein to minimize the effect of leptin.
- You might be eating too much fat. The keto is a fat based diet, but you cannot eat an unlimited amount of fat. Fat should be about 60 to 75% of your diet. Anything more will cause weight gain.
- If your body is already at a healthy natural level, then you will struggle to lose weight.
- Excessive exercise can block your fat loss goal because it increases appetite and leads to overeating.

Other things you should know

- Include omega-3 oils such as coconut oil, macadamia nuts and fatty fish to accelerate your fat loss.
- Only weigh yourself once weekly. No movement on weight scale doesn't mean you are gaining weight because muscles are heavier than fat. Don't only rely on scale, use body tape, belts, clothes, and calipers to see any changes.
- Avoid fat-free products.
- Eat only real, organic, whole foods.
- Be patient and continue with your diet.

CHAPTER 4

Frequently Asked Questions

In this chapter, we are going to discuss the frequently asked questions on Keto diet.

How long does it take to get into Ketosis?

It can take anywhere from 2 to 7 days to enter your body into Ketosis. The time depends on what you are eating, your activity levels and your body type. The easiest way to get into Ketosis is to limit your carb intake to 20g daily, exercise on an empty stomach and drinking plenty of water.

How to track my carb intake?

Search the internet and you will find plenty of good sites to track your carb intake.

What about eating too much fat?

Yes, you can eat too much fat. Search online and you will find plenty of Keto calculators that will help you calculate your macros and how much carb, proteins and fats you should consume in a day.

How much weight will I lose?

It depends on you. How many carbs you eat, your activity/exercise level determines how much weight you will lose.

How can I tell if I am in Ketosis?

Using Ketostix is an easy way to know if your body is in Ketosis or not. This device gives you a general idea if you are in Ketosis or not, but remember, they can be inaccurate. For a more reliable and accurate measurement, use blood ketone meter. You can find both Ketostix and blood Ketone meter on Amazon.

What about the risk of heart attacks because of the fats?

It was previously believed that saturated fats could cause heart disease, but recent research shows that saturated fats do not cause heart attacks, but improve cholesterol levels. Avoid vegetable oils and margarine spreads because they can cause heart disease. Polyunsaturated fats from fish are healthy. Monounsaturated fats are also healthy. So, basically, you only have to avoid trans fats, margarine spreads, and vegetable oils.

What are Macros and should I count them?

Macros are short for the world macronutrients. The main three macronutrients are carbohydrates, proteins, and fats. The best way to track your macros is thinking regarding grams.

- Fats are 10% anti-Ketogenic and 90% Ketogenic.
- Proteins are 58% anti-Ketogenic and 45% Ketogenic.
- Carbs are 100% anti-Ketogenic.

Keto Calculators will help you count your actual macros.

I just started the diet and I feel like it's not worth it

The initial symptoms of Keto diet can make things a bit difficult for a beginner like you. So drink plenty of water and broth. Eat salted nuts, deli meat, and bacon. These foods and drinks will keep you well balanced and functional.

Constipation problem

- Drink tea or coffee
- Eat chia and flax seeds
- Eat more fibrous vegetables
- Stop eating nuts
- Eat 1 tbsp. coconut oil
- Drink plenty of water
- Take a magnesium supplement

I am not losing weight anymore, what to do?

If you are not losing weight:

- Switch to measuring instead of weighing
- Avoid processed food
- Look for hidden carbs
- Avoid artificial sweeteners
- Stop eating gluten
- Stop eating nuts
- Lower your carb intake
- Increase your fat intake
- Cut out dairy

What about exercise?

If you do a lot of cardio like marathons, running and biking, then you don't have to worry because aerobic exercise isn't affected by carbohydrate diets. However, if you lift weights, then you need to eat more carb because carb helps your performance and help to gain muscles.

Supplements to take

Here are some common supplements you should take:

- Vitamin B Complex
- Vitamin D Supplement
- Potassium Supplement
- Magnesium Supplement
- Multivitamin for Men
- Multivitamin for Women

CHAPTER 5

Exercise During the Diet

The Ketogenic diet incorporates fat based food and nutrition because they are important to lose weight. The ketogenic diet gives you added benefits because you don't have to follow an extensive exercise routine to lose weight. But remember, aside fat loss, your aim should also include attaining better physical and mental health and muscle toning, which helps to increase your metabolism and accelerate weight loss.

Integrating exercise with keto promotes weight loss in many ways:

- Exercise increases insulin sensitivity of your body, boosts endorphin production, which reduces stress and lift mode. Studies reveal that stress is a crucial factor for weight gain. Lower levels of stress generally lead to a reduction in appetite and eventually help you to lose weight.
- Regular exercise will help you build body muscles and muscles stimulate fat burning. Body muscles boost your metabolic rate, and your body will burn more calories at a much quicker rate.

Developing your exercise program

According to guidelines, you need four types of fitness:

- **Flexibility:** Flexibility means you can move your body to do everything you need and want to do. Reduced flexibility can make your muscles work harder, cause pain and lead to injury.
- **Strength:** You need to exercise your body muscles to maintain their strength because inactive muscles become weak and shrink. Weak muscles make you feel weak, and you get tired quickly.
- **Aerobic:** Walking, swimming, running, dancing, riding a bike all are good examples of aerobic exercise. Aerobic exercise helps to control weight, improves cardiovascular fitness and lower heart attack risk.
- **Balance:** Good balance helps you prevent falling even when you age. Coordinated, strong leg and trunk muscles are an important part of your good balance.

Physical Activity Guidelines recommended by the U.S. Department of Health and Human Services

- Moderate endurance or aerobic exercise at least 2.5 hours (150 minutes) weekly or vigorous intensity activity for 75 minutes weekly.
- Aerobic exercise throughout the week, at least 10 minutes at a time.
- Moderate-intensity muscle-strengthening exercise for all main muscle groups at least 2 days weekly.
- If you can't follow the guidelines, then remain as active as possible.

Here are examples of 150 minutes of moderate-intensity aerobic exercise

- Moderate intensity 10-minute walk, three times daily, 5 days a week.

- Moderate intensity 20-minute bike ride, 3 days weekly. And a 30-minute walk, 3 days weekly.
- Moderate intensity 30-minute aerobic dance class, twice a week and three 10-minute walks, three days weekly.
- Gardening and yard work (lifting, raking, digging) 30 minutes a day, at least 5 days a week.

CHAPTER 6

Keto Diet Recipes

Breakfast Recipes

KETO EGG BUTTER WITH AVOCADO & SMOKED SALMON

Total Preparation & Cooking Time: 20 minutes
Servings: 2

Nutritional Value (Estimated Amount Per Serving)

Calories 1066	Cholesterol 537mg
Calories from Fat 935	Sodium 2325mg
Total Fat 104g	Potassium 959mg
Saturated Fat 45g	Total Carbohydrates 13g
Trans Fat 2.4g	Dietary Fiber 9.4g
Polyunsaturated Fat 8.5g	Sugars 0.8g
Monounsaturated Fat 43g	Protein 26g

Ingredients

- 5 oz. butter, at room temperature
- 4 oz. smoked salmon
- 2 avocados

- 4 eggs, large
- ¼ tsp. ground black pepper
- 1 tbsp. parsley, fresh & chopped
- 2 tbsp. olive oil
- ½ tsp. sea salt

Directions

1. Carefully place the eggs in a large-sized pot. Fill the pot with cold water (enough to cover the eggs by 1") & then place the pot on a stove, preferably without the lid. Bring it to a boil, over moderate heat settings.
2. Once starts boiling; decrease the heat settings & let simmer for 6 to 8 minutes. Carefully remove the eggs using a large spatula & place them in a bowl, preferably with cold water.
3. Once easy to handle; peel & finely chop the eggs. Now, using a large fork; mix eggs with the butter. Season the mixture with pepper, salt & any of your favorite flavors to taste.
4. Serve the egg butter with a side of diced avocado (preferably tossed in the olive oil) & few slices of smoked salmon and finely chopped parsley.

FRIED EGGS

Total Preparation & Cooking Time: 10 minutes
Servings: 4

Nutritional Value (Estimated Amount Per Serving)

Calories 245

Calories from Fat 189

Total Fat 21g

Saturated Fat 10g

Trans Fat 0.5g

Polyunsaturated Fat 2.3g

Monounsaturated Fat 6.6g

Cholesterol 402mg

Sodium 233mg

Potassium 141mg

Total Carbohydrates 0.7g

Dietary Fiber 0g

Sugars 0.4g

Protein 13g

Ingredients

- 2 oz. butter
- 8 eggs, large
- Pepper & salt to taste

Directions

1. Over moderate heat settings in a large frying pan; heat few tablespoons of coconut oil or butter until completely melted.
2. Now, crack the eggs in the middle of hot pan & fry them, preferably sunny side up. Sprinkle pepper & salt to taste. Serve warm & enjoy.

KETO BAKED BACON OMELET

Total Preparation & Cooking Time: 25 minutes
Servings: 1

Nutritional Value (Estimated Amount Per Serving)

Calories 1474

Calories from Fat 1185

Total Fat 132g

Saturated Fat 65g

Trans Fat 3g

Polyunsaturated Fat 14g

Monounsaturated Fat 45g

Cholesterol 705mg

Sodium 3273mg

Potassium 1186mg

Total Carbohydrates 5.6g

Dietary Fiber 1.4g

Sugars 0.7g

Protein 66g

Ingredients

- 2 oz. spinach, fresh
- 5 1/3 oz. bacon cubes
- 2 eggs, large
- 1 tbsp. chives, fresh & finely chopped
- 3 oz. butter
- Pepper & salt to taste

Directions

1. Lightly grease a large-sized baking dish with the butter and preheat your oven to 400 F in advance.
2. Fry spinach and bacon in the leftover butter.
3. Whisk the eggs for a minute or two, until completely frothy and then mix in the bacon & spinach.
4. Add some of the finely chopped chives and season with pepper and salt to taste.
5. Transfer the egg mixture into the baking dish & bake in

the preheated oven until set & turn golden brown, for 20 minutes.

6. Set aside and let cool for couple of minutes; serve & enjoy.

KETO CAULIFLOWER HASH WITH EGGS & POBLANO PEPPERS

Total Preparation & Cooking Time: 30 minutes
Servings: 2

Nutritional Value (Estimated Amount Per Serving)

Calories 454

Calories from Fat 398

Total Fat 44g

Saturated Fat 16g

Trans Fat 0.8g

Polyunsaturated Fat 14g

Monounsaturated Fat 12g

Cholesterol 243mg

Sodium 401mg

Potassium 287mg

Total Carbohydrates 6.7g

Dietary Fiber 3g

Sugars 3.2g

Protein 9.1g

Ingredients

- 4 eggs, large
- 1 pound cauliflower, grated
- 3 oz. butter
- 1 tsp. onion or garlic powder
- ½ cup mayonnaise
- 3 oz. Poblano peppers
- 1 tsp. olive oil
- Pepper & salt to taste

Directions

1. In a small-sized bowl; mix mayonnaise together with onion or garlic powder; mix well & set aside.
2. Using a food processor or a grater; chop or grate the cauliflower as well as the stem.

3. Now, over moderate heat settings in a large saucepan; heat the olive oil or butter & fry the grated cauliflower for couple of minutes. Season with pepper and salt to taste.
4. Brush a small amount of oil over the poblanos & grill or fry them until the skin begins to bubble.
5. Feel free to fry the eggs per your likings. Season with pepper and salt to taste. Serve directly with the cauliflower hash and roasted poblanos. Top the dish with a dollop of seasoned mayo.

KETO PANCAKES

Total Preparation & Cooking Time: 20 minutes
Servings: 1

Nutritional Value (Estimated Amount Per Serving)

Calories 503

Calories from Fat 385

Total Fat 43g

Saturated Fat 28g

Trans Fat 0.1g

Polyunsaturated Fat 3.1g

Monounsaturated Fat 8.4g

Cholesterol 390mg

Sodium 488mg

Potassium 178mg

Total Carbohydrates 3.8g

Dietary Fiber 1.5g

Sugars 1.3g

Protein 24g

Ingredients

- 2 tbsp. cashew milk, unsweetened
- 2/3 oz. pork rinds
- 1 tsp. maple extract
- 2 tbsp. coconut oil, for frying
- 1 tsp. ground cinnamon
- 2 eggs, large

Directions

1. Pulse the pork rinds over high settings in a blender until grounded into a fine powder. Add in the remaining ingredients & continue to combine until completely smooth.
2. Over moderate heat settings in a large skillet; heat a tbsp. of the coconut oil.
3. Pour approximately ¼ cup of batter into the hot skillet & fry for couple of minutes, until set & turn golden brown.

Flip & continue cooking until completely cooked through.

4. Remove from the skillet & repeat these steps with the leftover batter. Feel free to add more of coconut oil, if required.

KETO COCONUT PORRIDGE

Total Preparation & Cooking Time: 10 minutes
Servings: 1

Nutritional Value (Estimated Amount Per Serving)

Calories 586

Calories from Fat 396

Total Fat 44g

Saturated Fat 31g

Trans Fat 0.9g

Polyunsaturated Fat 2g

Monounsaturated Fat 8.5g

Cholesterol 247mg

Sodium 415mg

Potassium 189mg

Total Carbohydrates 42g

Dietary Fiber 1.3g

Sugars 40g

Protein 7.9g

Ingredients

- 1 tbsp. coconut flour
- A pinch of psyllium husk powder, ground
- 1 oz. butter
- 4 tbsp. coconut cream
- 1 egg, large
- A pinch of salt

Directions

1. Over low heat settings in a large-sized non-stick saucepan; mix all of the ingredients together; stirring frequently, until you get your desired texture.
2. Serve the Porridge with coconut cream or milk; topped with a few berries, fresh or frozen & enjoy.

KETO AVOCADO EGGS WITH BACON SAILS

Total Preparation & Cooking Time: 15 minutes
Servings: 4

Nutritional Value (Estimated Amount Per Serving)

Calories 143
Calories from Fat 102
Total Fat 11g
Saturated Fat 3g
Trans Fat 0g
Polyunsaturated Fat 1.6g
Monounsaturated Fat 5.7g
Cholesterol 107mg
Sodium 271mg
Potassium 188mg
Total Carbohydrates 2g
Dietary Fiber 1.2g
Sugars 0.3g
Protein 8.3g

Ingredients

- 2 oz. bacon
- ½ avocado
- 2 eggs, hard-boiled
- 1 tsp. olive oil
- Pepper & salt to taste

Directions

1. Carefully place the eggs in a large pot and then fill it water (enough to cover them by 1"). Hard boil the eggs, over moderate heat settings and let them cool a bit until easy to handle. Split the eggs (just like you do for the deviled eggs).
2. Scoop the yolk out & mash with the oil and avocado. Season with pepper and salt to taste.

3. Bake the bacon for 5 to 7 minutes, until crispy in a frying pan or at 350 F in the oven.
4. Carefully add the mixture again into the egg using a large spoon & set the bacon sail. Serve & enjoy.

KETO PANCAKES WITH BERRIES & WHIPPED CREAM

Total Preparation & Cooking Time: 30 minutes
Servings: 4

Nutritional Value (Estimated Amount Per Serving)

Calories 458

Calories from Fat 383

Total Fat 43g

Saturated Fat 28g

Trans Fat 0.8g

Polyunsaturated Fat 2.3g

Monounsaturated Fat 8.6g

Cholesterol 262mg

Sodium 267mg

Potassium 225mg

Total Carbohydrates 6.3g

Dietary Fiber 1.7g

Sugars 3.3g

Protein 14g

Ingredients

- 4 eggs, large
- 7 oz. cottage cheese
- 1 tbsp. ground psyllium husk powder
- 2 oz. coconut oil or butter

For Toppings:

- 1 cup heavy whipping cream
- 8 tbsp. blueberries or raspberries or strawberries, fresh

Directions

1. Using a large fork or spoon; blend all of the ingredients (except for toppings) in a large-sized bowl; set aside for couple of minutes and let the mixture to expand.
2. Now, over moderate heat settings in a large frying pan; heat oil or butter. Once hot; carefully place the pancakes &

fry them for 3 to 4 minutes per side. Carefully flip and cook the other side as well. Ensure you don't let the cottage cheese lumps to stick to the bottom of your pan.

3. Whip the heavy cream until soft peaks form. Serve the pancakes with some blueberries & whipped heavy cream.

KETO MEXICAN SCRAMBLED EGGS

Total Preparation & Cooking Time: 20 minutes
Servings: 4

Nutritional Value (Estimated Amount Per Serving)

Calories 253

Calories from Fat 181

Total Fat 20g

Saturated Fat 10g

Trans Fat 0.5g

Polyunsaturated Fat 2g

Monounsaturated Fat 6.2g

Cholesterol 315mg

Sodium 293mg

Potassium 222mg

Total Carbohydrates 3.1g

Dietary Fiber 0.7g

Sugars 1.6g

Protein 15g

Ingredients

- 6 eggs, large
- 2 tbsp. butter, for frying
- 1 scallion, fresh
- 3 oz. cheese, shredded
- 1 tomato, chopped finely
- 2 jalapeños, pickled, chopped finely
- Pepper & salt to taste

Directions

1. Over moderate heat settings in a large saucepan; heat the butter. Finely chop the tomatoes, jalapeños & scallions. Once you can see bubbles in the pan; fry the chopped tomatoes, jalapeños & scallions for 2 to 3 minutes.
2. Beat the eggs & pour into the middle of your pan. Scramble for a minute or two. Then add in the cheese & seasoning to taste. Serve warm & enjoy.

KETO MUSHROOM OMELET

Total Preparation & Cooking Time: 20 minutes
Servings: 1

Nutritional Value (Estimated Amount Per Serving)

Calories 563

Calories from Fat 423

Total Fat 47g

Saturated Fat 25g

Trans Fat 1.2g

Polyunsaturated Fat 4.2g

Monounsaturated Fat 14g

Cholesterol 647mg

Sodium 583mg

Potassium 442mg

Total Carbohydrates 8.6g

Dietary Fiber 1.5g

Sugars 3.8g

Protein 27g

Ingredients

- 1 oz. cheese, shredded
- 3 mushrooms
- 1 oz. butter, for frying
- 3 eggs, large
- ½ yellow onion, chopped
- Pepper & salt to taste

Directions

1. Crack the eggs in a large-sized mixing bowl & then sprinkle a pinch of each pepper & salt. Using a fork; whisk the eggs until completely smooth & frothy.
2. Add spices and salt to taste.
3. Over moderate heat settings in a large saucepan; heat the butter until completely melted. Pour the egg mixture in the middle of the hot pan & cook.
4. When the omelet get firm, but you can still see a little raw

egg on the top, sprinkle onion, cheese and mushrooms on top.

5. Carefully ease around the omelet's edges using a large spatula & then fold it in half. When it begins to turn golden brown, remove the pan from heat & carefully slide the cooked omelet on to a large-sized plate.

KETO CAPRESE OMELET

Total Preparation & Cooking Time: 20 minutes
Servings: 2

Nutritional Value (Estimated Amount Per Serving)

Calories 570	Cholesterol 618mg
Calories from Fat 403	Sodium 690mg
Total Fat 45g	Potassium 386mg
Saturated Fat 17g	Total Carbohydrates 4.7g
Trans Fat 0.1g	Dietary Fiber 0.6g
Polyunsaturated Fat 4.9g	Sugars 2.6g
Monounsaturated Fat 20g	Protein 36g

Ingredients

- 3 ½ oz. tomatoes, cut in slices or cherry tomatoes, cut in halves
- 6 eggs, large
- 5 1/3 oz. mozzarella cheese, fresh
- 1 tbsp. basil, fresh or dried
- 2 tbsp. olive oil
- Pepper & salt to taste

Directions

1. In a large-sized mixing bowl; crack the eggs and then add black pepper and salt to taste. Using a large fork; whisk until combined completely. Add in the basil; give everything a good stir.
2. Slice or dice the cheese and cut the tomatoes in slices or halves.
3. Over moderate heat settings in a large frying pan; heat the

oil & fry the tomatoes for couple of minutes.

4. Transfer the egg batter over the tomatoes. Wait for a minute or two, until the batter is firm slightly and then add the mozzarella cheese.

5. Decrease the heat settings & let it set completely. Serve immediately & enjoy.

KETO EGG MUFFINS

Total Preparation & Cooking Time: 30 minutes
Servings: 4

Nutritional Value (Estimated Amount Per Serving)

Calories 213

Calories from Fat 145

Total Fat 16g

Saturated Fat 6.7g

Trans Fat 0.2g

Polyunsaturated Fat 2.1g

Monounsaturated Fat 5.7g

Cholesterol 301mg

Sodium 264mg

Potassium 139mg

Total Carbohydrates 1.8g

Dietary Fiber 0.1g

Sugars 0.5g

Protein 15g

Ingredients

- 6 eggs, large
- 1 tbsp. green or red pesto
- 3 oz. cheese, shredded
- 1 scallion, chopped finely
- 5 oz. cooked bacon or salami or chorizo, air dried
- Pepper & salt to taste

Directions

1. Preheat your oven to 350 F in advance.
2. Finely chop the meat & scallions.
3. Whisk eggs together with pesto and seasoning. Add in the cheese; give everything a good stir.
4. Fill the muffin forms, preferably half with the batter & add bacon, salami or chorizo.
5. Bake in the preheated oven for 15 to 20 minutes.

CHICKEN, BACON, AVOCADO CAESAR SALAD

Total Preparation & Cooking Time: 20 minutes
Servings: 2

Nutritional Value (Estimated Amount Per Serving)

Calories 833	Cholesterol 169mg
Calories from Fat 551	Sodium 2145mg
Total Fat 61g	Potassium 1185mg
Saturated Fat 17g	Total Carbohydrates 9.8g
Trans Fat 0.2g	Dietary Fiber 5.7g
Polyunsaturated Fat 14g	Sugars 1.2g
Monounsaturated Fat 27g	Protein 59g

Ingredients

- 1 chicken breast, pre-cooked or grilled
- Lettuce, fresh
- 1 avocado, ripe & sliced
- Creamy Caesar dressing to taste
- 1 cup bacon, pre-cooked, crumbled (approximately 4 slices)

Directions

1. Slice the avocado in half, twist & discard the pit. Then again, slice in half and get rid of the shell. Slice it further into approximately 1-inch slices.
2. Slice the grilled/pre-cooked chicken breast into thin slices.
3. Combine avocado slices together with crumbled bacon &

chicken breast between two bowls.

4. Top the bowls with couple dollops of the Creamy Caesar dressing; toss lightly (don't swoosh the avocado).
5. Pour the salad over the lettuce.
6. Serve & enjoy.

FRESH SRIRACHA BROCCOLI SALAD

Total Preparation & Cooking Time: 15 minutes
Servings: 4

Nutritional Value (Estimated Amount Per Serving)

Calories 730

Calories from Fat 615

Total Fat 68g

Saturated Fat 13g

Trans Fat 0.3g

Polyunsaturated Fat 37g

Monounsaturated Fat 16g

Cholesterol 54mg

Sodium 2750mg

Potassium 720mg

Total Carbohydrates 15g

Dietary Fiber 6.6g

Sugars 3.7g

Protein 18g

Ingredients

- ½ cup cheddar cheese, shredded
- 1 – 1 ½ large heads broccoli, chopped (approximately 4 heaping cups)
- ½ tbsp. apple cider vinegar
- 1 cup mayonnaise
- ¼ to ½ tbsp. Sriracha sauce
- 6 slices of bacon, baked & crumbled
- ½ red bell pepper, cored, sliced & chopped into ¼" bites
- Freshly cracked black pepper & salt to taste
- ¼ cup salted sunflower seeds, dry roasted (shelled)

Directions

1. Mix the entire ingredients together in a large-sized bowl; give everything a good toss until evenly combined.
2. Store in an air-right container, preferably sealed for couple of hours. Serve & enjoy.

KETO GARLIC MASCARPONE BROCCOLI ALFREDO FRIED PIZZA

Total Preparation & Cooking Time: 30 minutes
Servings: 4

Nutritional Value (Estimated Amount Per Serving)

Calories 308

Calories from Fat 259

Total Fat 29g

Saturated Fat 17g

Trans Fat 0.3g

Polyunsaturated Fat 1.1g

Monounsaturated Fat 7.8g

Cholesterol 86mg

Sodium 461mg

Potassium 104mg

Total Carbohydrates 3g

Dietary Fiber 0.5g

Sugars 1.3g

Protein 11g

Ingredients

- 1 cup mozzarella cheese, shredded
- ¼ cup mascarpone cheese
- 1 tbsp. heavy cream
- 2 tbsp. ghee
- 1/3 cup broccoli heads, steamed & chopped
- 1 tsp. garlic, minced
- Asiago cheese, shaved to taste
- 1 cup pizza cheese blend, shredded
- 1/8 tsp. lemon pepper seasoning
- 1 tbsp. garlic olive oil
- Pinches of salt

Directions

1. Over medium heat settings in a large non-stick pan; heat the olive oil and wait until hot & starts shimmering.

2. First, add in the pizza cheese blend & form into a circle. Put the mozzarella cheese over the top & form into a circle again.
3. Cook until gets crispy & you are able to slide a spatula easily under the edges completely & are able to slide the crust onto a large-sized plate to cool, for 4 to 5 minutes.
4. Add in the ghee, mascarpone cheese, garlic, heavy cream, salt and lemon pepper to the pan; cook until begins to bubble and melted, then carefully remove the pan from heat; ensure you don't break it into pieces.
5. Drizzle half of the mixture on top of the crust. Add broccoli (chopped & steamed) to the other half.
6. Cook until hot & bubbling, for a minute more. Add broccoli to the pizza and finally sprinkle the Asiago cheese shavings & more of lemon pepper seasoning on the top.

SWEET SAUSAGE STUFFED BANANA PEPPERS

Total Preparation & Cooking Time: 30 minutes
Servings: 4

Nutritional Value (Estimated Amount Per Serving)

Calories 452	Cholesterol 106mg
Calories from Fat 317	Sodium 1084mg
Total Fat 35g	Potassium 831mg
Saturated Fat 12g	Total Carbohydrates 12g
Trans Fat 0.1g	Dietary Fiber 5g
Polyunsaturated Fat 6.5g	Sugars 5.8g
Monounsaturated Fat 14g	Protein 24g

Ingredients

- 4 banana peppers; chop the ends off & make a boat by slicing it down the middle
- ½ tsp. herbs de Provence
- 1 pound sweet sausage
- 3 tbsp. yellow onions, chopped
- 1 tbsp. ghee
- Marinara sauce

Directions

1. Preheat your oven to 350 F in advance.
2. Coat the banana peppers with olive oil & then place them inside the preheated oven for approximately 20 minutes.
3. Cook the sausage in a large saucepan; until crumbled, over medium heat settings.

4. Once cooked; add ghee, onions & Herbs de Provence.
5. Decrease the heat settings & cook for 4 to 5 more minutes, on low heat settings.
6. Remove the banana peppers from oven; turn the temperature of your broiler up to 500 F.
7. Fill the banana peppers with the sausage mixture and then top them with the mozzarella cheese.
8. Put a thin layer of marinara on top of the stuffed peppers and place it on a plate, preferably oven-safe; cook until mozzarella is hot & starts bubbling, for 5 to 10 more minutes. Serve immediately & enjoy.

BACON BLEU ZOODLE SALAD

Total Preparation & Cooking Time: 5 minutes
Servings: 2

Nutritional Value (Estimated Amount Per Serving)

Calories 603

Calories from Fat 432

Total Fat 48g

Saturated Fat 15g

Trans Fat 0.6g

Polyunsaturated Fat 15g

Monounsaturated Fat 16g

Cholesterol 85mg

Sodium 1552mg

Potassium 1426mg

Total Carbohydrates 15g

Dietary Fiber 5g

Sugars 7.8g

Protein 30g

Ingredients

- 1/3 cup bleu cheese dressing, thick/chunky
- 4 cups zucchini noodles
- ½ cup bacon, crumbled
- 1 cup spinach, fresh
- 1/3 cup bleu cheese, crumbled
- Cracked pepper, fresh to taste

Directions

1. Put everything together in a large-sized bowl; give everything a good toss until evenly combined. Serve & enjoy.

SUNDRIED TOMATO PISTACHIO & GOAT CHEESE BALLS

Total Preparation & Cooking Time: 20 minutes
Servings: 7

Nutritional Value (Estimated Amount Per Serving)

Calories 50	Cholesterol 0mg
Calories from Fat 36	Sodium 121mg
Total Fat 4g	Potassium 88mg
Saturated Fat 0.5g	Total Carbohydrates 2.4g
Trans Fat 0g	Dietary Fiber 0.9g
Polyunsaturated Fat 1.2g	Sugars 0.7g
Monounsaturated Fat 2.2g	Protein 1.8g

Ingredients

- ½ cup pistachios, de-shelled
- 1 package sundried tomato goat cheese (4-oz); cut into 7 slices & form into balls
- Salt to taste

Directions

1. Crush the pistachios lightly using a mortar & pestle (don't grind)
2. Sprinkle salt over the pistachio mixture.
3. Cover the goat cheese balls in the pistachio mixture; roll them.
4. Once completely coated, roll the balls again in the remaining pistachio dust
5. Serve & enjoy.

PESTO-MOZZARELLA FRIED PIZZA

Total Preparation & Cooking Time: 30 minutes
Servings: 4

Nutritional Value (Estimated Amount Per Serving)

Calories 111

Calories from Fat 80

Total Fat 8.8g

Saturated Fat 3.7g

Trans Fat 0g

Polyunsaturated Fat 0.9g

Monounsaturated Fat 3.5g

Cholesterol 20mg

Sodium 288mg

Potassium 96mg

Total Carbohydrates 2.3g

Dietary Fiber 0.4g

Sugars 1g

Protein 6.1g

Ingredients

- 1/3 cup low-carb tomato sauce
- 1 ½ cups mozzarella cheese
- Parmesan cheese, grated to taste
- 1 tbsp. garlic infused olive oil
- Italian/pizza seasonings to taste

For Toppings:

- 2 mozzarella balls, small & sliced into 4 slices
- 2 tbsp. pesto
- ¼ cup mozzarella cheese

Directions

1. Preheat the broiler to 500 F in advance.
2. Over medium heat settings in a large-sized, non-stick pan; heat the garlic oil. Swirl to coat the pan entirely and then add in the mozzarella.

3. Evenly spread the cheese using a large spatula, just like you do for a pizza. Cook until it starts to melt & turn dark around the edges, for 3 to 5 minutes.
4. Once the entire cheese starts to brown and has melted, add in the tomato sauce; lightly spread around the edges using a large spoon. Cook for a minute or two.
5. Start sliding it around the edges using a large spatula & then underneath (don't try to lift it out from the pan and ensure it doesn't stick to the bottom).
6. Now, tip your pan using a large spatula & slide the pizza on to a pan lined with an aluminum foil
7. Sprinkle grated cheese followed by the pizza seasonings over the top. Top with a few dollops of pesto, ¼ cup of mozzarella & mozzarella slices.
8. Place in the preheated oven until toppings are hot, for a minute or two.
9. Let sit for couple of minutes at room temperature & then cut into fours
10. Serve immediately & enjoy.

BUTTER COFFEE RUBBED TRI-TIP STEAK

Total Preparation & Cooking Time: 45 minutes
Servings: 2

Nutritional Value (Estimated Amount Per Serving)

Calories 1332	Cholesterol 472mg
Calories from Fat 689	Sodium 2050mg
Total Fat 77g	Potassium 1943mg
Saturated Fat 1.9g	Total Carbohydrates 2.6g
Trans Fat 0g	Dietary Fiber 0.6g
Polyunsaturated Fat 1.4g	Sugars 0.1g
Monounsaturated Fat 9.9g	Protein 149g

Ingredients

- 1 tsp. course ground black pepper
- 2 Tri-tip steaks or any beef cuts
- 1 package Coffee Blocks
- ½ tbsp. garlic powder
- 2 tbsp. olive oil
- ½ tbsp. sea salt

Directions

1. Let the meat to sit for several minutes at room temperature.
2. Combine the entire ingredients (except the steaks) in a large-sized bowl.
3. Coat all sides of the steaks with this mixture.
4. Now, over medium-high heat settings in a large skillet; heat the olive oil & cook the coated steaks for approximately 5 minutes per side.

5. Flip & cook the other side until the internal temperature reaches 140 F, for 5 more minutes.
6. Remove the pan from heat & let sit for couple of minutes, until it absorbs its own juices.
7. Cut the cooked steak against the grain into slices; serve & enjoy.

KETO SLOW-COOKER BEEF & BROCCOLI

Total Preparation & Cooking Time: 40 minutes
Servings: 4

Nutritional Value (Estimated Amount Per Serving)

Calories 459

Calories from Fat 173

Total Fat 19g

Saturated Fat 7.8g

Trans Fat 0g

Polyunsaturated Fat 0.9g

Monounsaturated Fat 7.7g

Cholesterol 179mg

Sodium 646mg

Potassium 891mg

Total Carbohydrates 3.6g

Dietary Fiber 0.8g

Sugars 1.4g

Protein 64g

Ingredients

- 1 cup beef broth
- 2 pounds flank steak; sliced into 1-2" chunks
- 1 tsp. ginger, freshly grated
- 2/3 cup liquid aminos such as Braggs or coconut aminos
- 3 tbsp. Stevia sweetener
- 1 red bell pepper
- ¼ - ½ tsp. red pepper flakes
- 1 head of broccoli, large
- 3 cloves garlic, minced
- 1 tsp. sesame seeds
- ½ tsp. salt or to taste

Directions

1. Preheat your slow cooker over low heat settings.
2. Place the sliced steak in the bottom of your slow cooker and then add in the beef broth, aminos, red pepper flakes, garlic cloves, ginger, sweetener & salt.
3. Cook for 5 to 6 hours on low heat settings.
4. In the meantime; prepare the red bell pepper & broccoli. Slice red bell pepper into 1" pieces, preferably large-sized & chop the broccoli into small florets.
5. Once the cooking cycle completes; give everything a good stir.
6. Transfer the red bell pepper and broccoli over the top until you get your desired crispness, for a minimum period of an hour, toss them together.
7. Sprinkle sesame seeds over the top. Serve & enjoy.

GARLIC BOMB PARMESAN WINGS

Total Preparation & Cooking Time: 40 minutes
Servings: 4

Nutritional Value (Estimated Amount Per Serving)

Calories 549	Cholesterol 131mg
Calories from Fat 356	Sodium 1373mg
Total Fat 40g	Potassium 293mg
Saturated Fat 15g	Total Carbohydrates 18g
Trans Fat 0.5g	Dietary Fiber 0.7g
Polyunsaturated Fat 6.4g	Sugars 0.4g
Monounsaturated Fat 14g	Protein 30g

Ingredients

- 20 wing sections, frozen (drums and wings)
- 1 cup Parmesan, grated
- 2 tbsp. garlic infused olive oil
- 1 tsp. garlic salt
- ½ tbsp. garlic powder

Directions

1. Preheat your oven to 450 F in advance.
2. Place the frozen wings on top of a baking pan, preferably on the roasting/baking rack. Sprinkle garlic salt over the top.
3. Cook until the thermometer reflects 180 F, for 35 minutes. Baste the wings with 1 tbsp. or more of garlic oil.
4. Broil for 5 minutes until skin is crispy & turn brown. Remove from oven & place it in a large-sized bowl.
5. Pour a tbsp. more of garlic oil; toss until evenly coated. Toss with grated Parmesan & garlic powder. Serve & enjoy.

LEMON THYME CHICKEN ON ROSEMARY SKEWERS

Total Preparation & Cooking Time: 1 hour & 10 minutes
Servings: 2

Nutritional Value (Estimated Amount Per Serving)

Calories 392	Cholesterol 191mg
Calories from Fat 81	Sodium 170mg
Total Fat 9g	Potassium 636mg
Saturated Fat 2.7g	Total Carbohydrates 3.9g
Trans Fat 0g	Dietary Fiber 2.6g
Polyunsaturated Fat 1.9g	Sugars 0g
Monounsaturated Fat 3g	Protein 70g

Ingredients

- 10 chicken tenderloins (approximately 1 ½ pounds)
- ½ tbsp. of each lemon pepper seasoning, garlic salt & rosemary or regular olive oil
- A few sprigs of thyme, fresh
- 10 rosemary skewers, preferably 6" (soaked in water for a minimum period of an hour)

Directions

1. Preheat your oven to 350 F in advance.
2. Waddle a point on the end of each stick using a short and sharp knife.
3. Toss the meat with the leftover ingredients in a large-sized bowl. Now, sprinkle the leaves of thyme.
4. Skewer each coated chicken tenderloin with a rosemary stick and bake in the preheated oven for 40 minutes.
5. Serve warm & enjoy.

BUFFALO PULLED CHICKEN & BLEU CHEESE WEDGE

Total Preparation & Cooking Time: 50 minutes
Servings: 2

Nutritional Value (Estimated Amount Per Serving)

Calories 434	Cholesterol 133mg
Calories from Fat 179	Sodium 2906mg
Total Fat 20g	Potassium 1346mg
Saturated Fat 6.3g	Total Carbohydrates 13g
Trans Fat 0.1g	Dietary Fiber 6.9g
Polyunsaturated Fat 5.1g	Sugars 5.1g
Monounsaturated Fat 6.8g	Protein 51g

Ingredients

- 4 bacon strips, uncured & nitrate-free
- 2 boneless chicken breasts
- Bleu cheese dressing
- 1 head of lettuce
- 2 tbsp. bleu cheese, crumbled
- ¾ cup buffalo sauce

Directions

1. Fill a large pot with water and add a small amount of salt to it. Bring it to a boil over moderate heat settings.
2. Once boiling; add in the chicken breasts & let cook until a meat thermometer reflects the internal temperature of the meat as 180 F, for half an hour.
3. Carefully remove the chicken pieces & cool for 10 to 12 minutes.

4. Meanwhile, cook the bacon strips in the microwave until cooked well, for 5 minutes.
5. Wash the lettuce under cold and running tap water.
6. Remove the bottom & then cut the lettuce in half; begin from the top towards the root.
7. Arrange two of the lettuce wedges on two large-sized plates.
8. When the bacon is cooked, put it inside a refrigerator and let it cool.
9. Pull the chicken apart into strips using a large fork (in the same manner which you would do with the pork).
10. Add the chicken to a small-sized pot, preferably over medium heat settings on the stove.
11. Top the chicken with the buffalo sauce; give everything a good stir & cook the chicken until hot.
12. Top the lettuce wedges with the bleu cheese dressing, you need to choose the amount of the dressing.
13. Top the dressing with some of the blue cheese crumbles
14. Remove the bacon from the fridge; crumbling it over the two wedges.
15. Add the buffalo pulled chicken to the plates & top with additional bleu cheese crumbles. Serve & enjoy.

GARLIC CAULIFLOWER BREADSTICKS

Total Preparation & Cooking Time: 50 minutes
Servings: 2

Nutritional Value (Estimated Amount Per Serving)

Calories 298
Calories from Fat 195
Total Fat 22g
Saturated Fat 12g
Trans Fat 0.3g
Polyunsaturated Fat 1.2g
Monounsaturated Fat 6.3g

Cholesterol 155mg
Sodium 648mg
Potassium 407mg
Total Carbohydrates 8.4g
Dietary Fiber 2.2g
Sugars 2.7g
Protein 19g

Ingredients

- 3 tsp. garlic, minced
- 1 tbsp. butter, organic
- ½ tsp. Italian seasoning
- 2 cups cauliflower rice; cooked for 3 minutes in the microwave
- 1 egg, large
- ¼ tsp. red pepper flakes
- Parmesan cheese, grated
- 1 cup mozzarella cheese, shredded
- 1/8 tsp. kosher salt

Directions

1. Preheat your oven to 350 F in advance.
2. Over low heat settings in a small-sized pan; melt the butter. Add red pepper flakes and garlic to the butter; cook for couple of minutes (make sure that the butter is not brown).

3. Place the cooked cauliflower rice to a large-sized bowl. Add the butter & garlic mixture to the bowl with cooked cauliflower rice.
4. Add salt and Italian seasoning to the bowl; mix well. Refrigerate for couple of minutes. Add the mozzarella cheese and egg to the bowl; mix again.
5. Cover the bottom of a baking dish, preferably 9×9"with a layer of parchment paper & lightly grease it up using cooking spray or butter. Add egg and mozzarella to the cauliflower mixture.
6. Add to your pan and using your palms; smooth the mixture into a thin layer. Bake in the preheated oven for half an hour.
7. Remove from the oven & top with some of the powdered parmesan (preferably few shakes) and additional mozzarella cheese.
8. Cook for 6 to 8 more minutes. Remove from oven & then cut into sticks. Serve & enjoy.

KETO BUFFALO WINGS

Total Preparation & Cooking Time: 30 minutes
Servings: 3

Nutritional Value (Estimated Amount Per Serving)

Calories 1005

Calories from Fat 655

Total Fat 73g

Saturated Fat 27g

Trans Fat 0.9g

Polyunsaturated Fat 13g

Monounsaturated Fat 30g

Cholesterol 520mg

Sodium 957mg

Potassium 767mg

Total Carbohydrates 1.2g

Dietary Fiber 0.3g

Sugars 0.3g

Protein 81g

Ingredients

- 12 chicken wings
- ¼ cup Frank's hot sauce
- 1 garlic clove, minced
- 4 tbsp. butter
- A grind of pepper, fresh
- ¼ tsp. of each paprika, cayenne pepper & salt

Directions

1. Bake the chicken wings and add butter & garlic to a microwave-safe bowl.
2. Heat the garlic and butter mixture up in the microwave.
3. Once the butter is melted, add the remaining ingredients; mix them all together.
4. The moment your wings are cooked through, toss them with the garlic-butter mixture in a bowl until evenly coated. Serve & enjoy.

LEMON PEPPER PULLED CHICKEN

Total Preparation & Cooking Time: 40 minutes
Servings: 6

Nutritional Value (Estimated Amount Per Serving)

Calories 547	Cholesterol 218mg
Calories from Fat 206	Sodium 1548mg
Total Fat 23g	Potassium 628mg
Saturated Fat 8.6g	Total Carbohydrates 8.2g
Trans Fat 0.4g	Dietary Fiber 0.9g
Polyunsaturated Fat 3.1g	Sugars 0.1g
Monounsaturated Fat 9.1g	Protein 73g

Ingredients

- 2-3 pounds chicken tenderloins
- 1 tbsp. lemon pepper
- ½ butter stick, organic
- Slices of cheddar cheese
- 1 tsp. thyme, dried
- 2 tbsp. olive/grape-seed oil
- Dijon mustard
- 1 tbsp. cloves garlic, minced
- Wrap of your choice
- 1 tbsp. adobo seasoned salt

Directions

1. Throw butter together with oil, garlic cloves, lemon pepper, thyme and seasoned salt into the bottom of your crockpot. Cook on high heat settings until fragrant & the butter is completely melted.

2. Now, place the chicken pieces in the crock pot; give everything a good stir and ensure that the chicken is entirely coated in the butter and seasonings.
3. Cook on high heat settings for 4 hours or for 6 hours on low heat settings, until the chicken easily pulls apart.
4. Once done, using a fork; shred the chicken inside the crockpot & mix with the juice; let the chicken to soak up the flavor completely. Let sit on low heat settings for 10 to 15 minutes, preferably in the juices.
5. Serve & enjoy. You can also store the leftovers in a fridge for dinner.

CHEESY KALE CASSEROLE

Total Preparation & Cooking Time: 30 minutes
Servings: 4

Nutritional Value (Estimated Amount Per Serving)

Calories 499	Cholesterol 122mg
Calories from Fat 256	Sodium 1468mg
Total Fat 28g	Potassium 1136mg
Saturated Fat 9.9g	Total Carbohydrates 18g
Trans Fat 0.6g	Dietary Fiber 4.2g
Polyunsaturated Fat 2.5g	Sugars 8.1g
Monounsaturated Fat 13g	Protein 42g

Ingredients

- 1 pound lean ground beef
- 2 cups marinara sauce
- 1 tsp. oregano
- 4 oz. mozzarella, shredded
- 1 tsp. garlic powder
- 10 oz. kale, fresh
- 1 tsp. onion powder
- ½ tsp. black pepper
- 2 tbsp. olive oil
- 1 tsp. kosher salt

Directions

1. Preheat your broiler over high heat settings.
2. Over medium-high heat settings in a Dutch oven or an

oven & broiler-safe deep skillet, heat the olive oil for couple of minutes.

3. Once hot; carefully place the beef & cook for 5 to 7 minutes, until no longer raw, stirring to crumble & break up the beef.

4. Add garlic powder, pepper, salt, oregano and onion powder; give everything a good stir. Work in batches & stir in the kale; cook until just wilts slightly.

5. Add the marinara sauce; give everything a good stir. Cook for couple of more minutes, until heated through. Add half of the cheese into the mixture; mix well.

6. Transfer the mixture to a dish (preferably broiler-safe), if you are not using the oven-safe skillet. Sprinkle the leftover cheese over the top. Broil for a minute, until cheese is just melted. Let rest for 5 minutes, before serving. Serve & enjoy.

EASY CASHEW CHICKEN

Total Preparation & Cooking Time: 25 minutes
Servings: 3

Nutritional Value (Estimated Amount Per Serving)

Calories 408	Cholesterol 137mg
Calories from Fat 263	Sodium 759mg
Total Fat 29g	Potassium 484mg
Saturated Fat 5.3g	Total Carbohydrates 8.6g
Trans Fat 0.1g	Dietary Fiber 1.3g
Polyunsaturated Fat 8.1g	Sugars 1.7g
Monounsaturated Fat 15g	Protein 31g

Ingredients

- 3 boneless, skinless chicken thighs, raw; dice into 1" chunks
- 1 tbsp. rice wine vinegar
- ¼ cup cashews
- 1 ½ tbsp. soy sauce
- 1 tbsp. Sesame Oil
- ½ tbsp. garlic-chili sauce
- 1 tbsp. garlic, minced
- ¼ white onion, medium & cut into equally large chunks
- 1 tbsp. Sesame Seeds
- ½ tsp. ground ginger
- 1 tbsp. green onions
- ½ Green Bell Pepper, medium & cut into equally large chunks
- 2 tbsp. canola oil
- Pepper & salt to taste

Directions

1. Over low heat settings in a large pan; toast the cashews until become fragrant & start to turn brown lightly, for 8 minutes. Remove & set aside.
2. Increase the heat settings to high & heat the canola oil.
3. Once hot, carefully place the chicken thighs & cook them for 5 minutes, until cooked through.
4. Once the chicken is completely cooked through; add in the onions, pepper, chili garlic sauce, garlic & seasonings (pepper, ginger & salt). Cook for couple of more minutes on high heat settings.
5. Add in the rice wine vinegar, soy sauce & the roasted cashews. Cook until it gets a sticky consistency & the liquid is reduced down, over high heat settings.
6. Transfer everything in a large-sized bowl & top the bowl with some of the sesame seeds; drizzle sesame oil over the top. Serve & enjoy.

BUNLESS BURGER

Total Preparation & Cooking Time: 20 minutes
Servings: 2

Nutritional Value (Estimated Amount Per Serving)

Calories 285	Cholesterol 73mg
Calories from Fat 169	Sodium 1594mg
Total Fat 19g	Potassium 451mg
Saturated Fat 8.2g	Total Carbohydrates 6.4g
Trans Fat 0.7g	Dietary Fiber 2.6g
Polyunsaturated Fat 0.9g	Sugars 2.1g
Monounsaturated Fat 6.9g	Protein 23g

Ingredients

- 4 ground beef patties (approximately ¼ pounds)
- 2 thick slices of tomato
- 12 tsp. Dijon mustard
- 2 slices of red onion
- 4 lettuce leaves
- ½ tsp. black pepper
- 2 sharp cheddar slices
- ½ tsp. coarse kosher salt

Directions

1. Generously season the beef patties with pepper & salt. Cook them for couple of minutes on each side on a hot cast iron griddle. Transfer them to a large-sized plate & let rest for couple of minutes, loosely covered in an aluminum foil.
2. In the meantime, assemble the leftover ingredients.

3. Grab two plates for sandwiches. Place 1 cooked patty on each of the plates. Spread mustard over the top of the patties. Layer the lettuce, cheese, tomato & onion on top of the mustard and then top with one more cooked patty.
4. Serve immediately & enjoy.

GARLIC ROASTED SHRIMP WITH ZUCCHINI PASTA

Total Preparation & Cooking Time: 20 minutes
Servings: 2

Nutritional Value (Estimated Amount Per Serving)

Calories 409	Cholesterol 272mg
Calories from Fat 261	Sodium 1375mg
Total Fat 29g	Potassium 810mg
Saturated Fat 11g	Total Carbohydrates 10g
Trans Fat 0g	Dietary Fiber 2.6g
Polyunsaturated Fat 2.9g	Sugars 4g
Monounsaturated Fat 14g	Protein 29g

Ingredients

- 2 tbsp. olive oil
- 8 ounces shrimp, peeled & deveined; thawed, if using frozen
- 2 zucchini, medium & spiralized or sliced into thin strips
- Zest & juice of 1 lemon
- 2 cloves garlic minced
- Freshly ground pepper to taste
- 2 tbsp. ghee melted
- ¼ tsp. salt

Directions

1. Preheat your oven to 400 F in advance.
2. Combine the entire ingredients (except the zucchini pasta)

in large-sized baking dish.

3. Bake in the preheated oven until shrimp are just cooked through and turns pink, for 8 to 10 minutes, turning once.

4. Add in the zucchini pasta; give everything a good toss to combine. Serve & enjoy.

TANDOORI SALMON

Total Preparation & Cooking Time: 15 minutes
Servings: 4

Nutritional Value (Estimated Amount Per Serving)

Calories 245   Cholesterol 71mg
Calories from Fat 130   Sodium 381mg
Total Fat 14g   Potassium 504mg
Saturated Fat 2.8g   Total Carbohydrates 2.3g
Trans Fat 0g   Dietary Fiber 1.1g
Polyunsaturated Fat 5.3g   Sugars 0.2g
Monounsaturated Fat 4.9g   Protein 26g

Ingredients

- 1 pound Salmon, wild-caught
- 2 tsp. paprika
- ¼ tsp. black pepper
- 1 tsp. garlic powder
- ½ tsp. garam masala
- 1 tsp. coriander powder
- ½ tsp. turmeric
- 3 tsp. mustard oil
- ¼ tsp. ginger powder
- 1 tsp. Kashmiri chili powder
- ½ tsp. salt

Directions

1. Line a large-sized baking sheet with an aluminum foil and preheat your oven to 425 F in advance.
2. Combine the entire spices together in a medium-sized

bowl; mix well. Add mustard oil; continue to mix until you get a paste like consistency.

3. Using your fingers; rub this paste over the salmon, preferably all sides.
4. Place the coated salmon, preferably skin-side down on the baking sheet, then place it inside the preheated oven.
5. Bake until the fish flakes easily, for 4 to 6 minutes per ½" thickness. Serve & enjoy.

CHILI ROASTED CHICKEN THIGHS

Total Preparation & Cooking Time: 20 minutes
Servings: 4

Nutritional Value (Estimated Amount Per Serving)

Calories 528

Calories from Fat 315

Total Fat 35g

Saturated Fat 9.9g

Trans Fat 0.2g

Polyunsaturated Fat 8g

Monounsaturated Fat 17g

Cholesterol 290mg

Sodium 598mg

Potassium 645mg

Total Carbohydrates 3.4g

Dietary Fiber 1.3g

Sugars 0.4g

Protein 54g

Ingredients

- Fresh ground pepper to taste
- 2 pounds chicken thighs, boneless
- Fresh cilantro for garnish
- 1 tbsp. chili powder
- Lime wedges for serving
- 1 tbsp. organic extra virgin olive oil
- Sea salt to taste

Directions

1. Preheat your oven to 375 F in advance.
2. Place the chicken thighs on a sheet pan & drizzle olive oil; turn several times until evenly coated with the oil. Now, rub the chicken pieces with chili powder, pepper, and salt.
3. Roast the chicken thighs for 12 to 15 minutes, until cooked through.
4. Sprinkle with fresh cilantro & serve with some lime wedges.

COCONUT CHICKEN TENDERS

Total Preparation & Cooking Time: 30 minutes
Servings: 4

Nutritional Value (Estimated Amount Per Serving)

Calories 502

Calories from Fat 304

Total Fat 34g

Saturated Fat 16g

Trans Fat 0.2g

Polyunsaturated Fat 9.4g

Monounsaturated Fat 5.4g

Cholesterol 99mg

Sodium 1078mg

Potassium 505mg

Total Carbohydrates 27g

Dietary Fiber 4.6g

Sugars 1.9g

Protein 24g

Ingredients

- ½ cup cashew flour
- 1 pound chicken tenders, boneless, skinless
- ¼ tsp. pepper
- 1 egg, large
- ¼ tsp. garlic powder
- ⅛ tsp. of cinnamon
- 1 cup coconut, unsweetened & shredded
- ¼ tsp. salt

Directions

1. Preheat your oven to 375 F in advance
2. Beat the egg in a medium-sized bowl; beat well & set aside.
3. Thoroughly combine the cashew flour with coconut & spices in a separate dish or bowl.
4. Lightly dip each piece of chicken tender first into the egg & then into the batter.

5. Arrange the coated chicken tenders on a large-sized baking sheet; lined either with a parchment paper or an aluminum foil.
6. Bake in the preheated oven until turns golden brown & no longer pink inside, for 15 to 20 minutes.

ROSEMARY APPLE PORK CHOPS

Total Preparation & Cooking Time: 35 minutes
Servings: 2

Nutritional Value (Estimated Amount Per Serving)

Calories 911

Calories from Fat 489

Total Fat 54g

Saturated Fat 15g

Trans Fat 0.4g

Polyunsaturated Fat 6.4g

Monounsaturated Fat 26g

Cholesterol 301mg

Sodium 216mg

Potassium 1302mg

Total Carbohydrates 8g

Dietary Fiber 1.4g

Sugars 4.9g

Protein 92g

Ingredients

For Pork Chops:

- 4 pork chops
- ½ apple
- 4 sprigs of rosemary, fresh
- 2 tbsp. olive oil
- Pepper, paprika & salt to taste

For Apple Cider Vinaigrette:

- 2 tbsp. olive oil
- 1 tbsp. lemon juice, freshly squeezed
- 2 tbsp. apple cider vinegar
- 1 tbsp. maple syrup, sugar-free
- Pepper & salt to taste

Directions

1. Heat up a large-sized cast iron skillet in a 400 F oven and prepare the pork chops.
2. Place each pork chop on a paper towel; pat them dry & rub them first with the olive oil and then with the seasonings. Remove the cast iron skillet from the oven & set it on high heat settings on the stove. Sear the pork chop, preferably each side for couple of minutes.
3. Lay the rosemary sprigs and apple slices over the pork chops & places them in the oven; cook until the internal temperature reaches 140 F, for 10 minutes.
4. In the meantime, prepare the apple cider vinaigrette by combining the entire ingredients together in a large bowl. Make sure you add the olive oil in the last. Slowly transfer it; continue to whisk the remaining vinaigrette. Once you have cooked the pork chops, pour the prepared vinaigrette on the top. Serve & enjoy.

EASY BUFFALO WINGS

Total Preparation & Cooking Time: 30 minutes
Servings: 2

Nutritional Value (Estimated Amount Per Serving)

Calories 108

Calories from Fat 106

Total Fat 12g

Saturated Fat 7.3g

Trans Fat 0.5g

Polyunsaturated Fat 0.5g

Monounsaturated Fat 3g

Cholesterol 31mg

Sodium 1598mg

Potassium 85mg

Total Carbohydrates 1g

Dietary Fiber 0.2g

Sugars 0.7g

Protein 0.4g

Ingredients

- 6 chicken wings or wingettes or drumettes
- 2 tbsp. butter
- ½ cup Frank's Red Hot Sauce
- Pepper, salt, garlic powder, cayenne & paprika to taste

Directions

1. Break up your chicken wings into two even-sized pieces (the drumettes & wingettes, discarding the tips). Put a small amount of the Frank's Red Hot sauce on top of the wings; make sure that all sides are coated evenly with the sauce.
2. Season the wings & toss them several times to cover them. Let refrigerate for an hour.
3. Turn on your broiler to high heat settings & place the oven rack approximately 6" from the broiler. Line a large-sized baking sheet with an aluminum foil. Lay the chicken

wings out; making sure that they have enough of space between them.

4. Cook them in the preheated broiler until the tops of the wings turn dark brown, for 8 to 10 minutes. Don't worry if some the tops turn black.

5. In the meantime, melt approximately 2 tbsp. of the butter & the remaining hot sauce. Lightly season it with the cayenne pepper. Once melted, remove it from the heat source.

6. Remove the cooked wings from the broiler; flip & place them again in the broiler for 6 to 8 more minutes. Don't let them burn.

7. Once all sides are cooked through, place them in a deep-sized mixing bowl & transfer the prepared hot sauce on top of them. Toss several times until evenly coated with the sauce. Enjoy them with some keto cole slaw, carrots, celery & bleu cheese.

PAN SEARED SALMON WITH SAUTÉED MUSHROOMS & SPINACH

Total Preparation & Cooking Time: 20 minutes
Servings: 2

Nutritional Value (Estimated Amount Per Serving)

Calories 779

Calories from Fat 487

Total Fat 54g

Saturated Fat 15g

Trans Fat 0.5g

Polyunsaturated Fat 13g

Monounsaturated Fat 22g

Cholesterol 174mg

Sodium 362mg

Potassium 2216mg

Total Carbohydrates 16g

Dietary Fiber 7.3g

Sugars 5.5g

Protein 59g

Ingredients

- 2 salmon fillets
- ½ pound mushrooms; sliced
- 2 cups spinach
- 2 Campari tomatoes; sliced
- 2 tbsp. butter
- 1 tbsp. balsamic vinegar
- 2 tbsp. olive oil (1 plus 1 tbsp.)
- Pepper & salt to taste
- 2 garlic cloves; sliced

Directions

1. Get rid of any excess moisture from the salmon fillets by placing them on paper towels; pat them dry. Generously season with pepper & salt, preferably both sides; keep

them inside a refrigerator fridge and prepare the remaining recipe.

2. Over medium heat settings in a large saucepan; heat 1 tbsp. of olive oil & cook the mushrooms and garlic for couple of minutes, until shrunken in size. This is the time to add in the butter.

3. Add in the tomatoes; wait for a minute or two and then add spinach in the last; cook for couple of minutes, until just wilted. Season with pepper and salt; toss well. Remove the veggies from heat and place them on a large plate. Using an aluminum foil; cover the plate and cook the salmon.

4. Now, in the same pan; heat one more tbsp. of olive oil until very hot.

5. Carefully lay the salmon fillets in the middle of your pan, preferably skin side down; sear them for 4 to 5 minutes. Ensure you don't move them around.

6. Flip and cook the other side of the fillets for 4 to 5 more minutes.

7. Lastly, uncover the veggies & drizzle them with some of the balsamic vinegar. Carefully place the cooked salmon fillets over the cooked veggies & garnish them with fresh lemon. Serve & enjoy.

DELICIOUS SESAME CHICKEN

Total Preparation & Cooking Time: 30 minutes
Servings: 2

Nutritional Value (Estimated Amount Per Serving)

Calories 597

Calories from Fat 339

Total Fat 38g

Saturated Fat 11g

Trans Fat 0.2g

Polyunsaturated Fat 9.6g

Monounsaturated Fat 17g

Cholesterol 383mg

Sodium 1311mg

Potassium 729mg

Total Carbohydrates 8.1g

Dietary Fiber 1.3g

Sugars 0.6g

Protein 59g

Ingredients

For Coating & Chicken:

- 1 pound chicken thighs, cut into bite-sized pieces
- 1 tbsp. corn starch or arrowroot powder
- 1 egg, large
- 1 tbsp. sesame seed oil, toasted
- Pepper & salt to taste

For Sesame Sauce:

- 2 tbsp. Sukrin Gold
- 1 tbsp. sesame seed oil, toasted
- 2 tbsp. soy sauce
- 1 cm ginger, cube
- 2 tbsp. sesame seeds
- 1 garlic clove
- ¼ tsp. xanthan gum
- 1 tbsp. vinegar

Directions

1. Combine egg together with a tbsp. of the arrowroot powder or corn starch & prepare the batter; whisk well & add in the pieces of chicken thigh. Turn several times into the mixture until all sides are evenly coated.
2. In the meantime; over moderate heat settings in a large saucepan; heat up a tbsp. of toasted sesame seed oil & cook the coated chicken thighs; leaving some room between each other. Work in batches & fry the chicken thighs for 10 minutes, if required; gently flipping & moving the chicken.
3. While you are cooking the chicken thighs. Now, combine the entire sauce ingredients in a large-bowl and prepare the sauce; whisk well.
4. When you have cooked the entire chicken pieces, add the sesame sauce to the pan; give everything a good stir until evenly combined & cook for 5 more minutes.
5. When the sauce has warmed up and thickened; remove the chicken pieces and transfer them to the bed of cooked broccoli. Sprinkle with more of sesame seeds & green onion. Serve & enjoy.

LEMON ROSEMARY CHICKEN THIGHS

Total Preparation & Cooking Time: 50 minutes
Servings: 2

Nutritional Value (Estimated Amount Per Serving)

Calories 677

Calories from Fat 429

Total Fat 48g

Saturated Fat 18g

Trans Fat 0.7g

Polyunsaturated Fat 9g

Monounsaturated Fat 20g

Cholesterol 363mg

Sodium 545mg

Potassium 743mg

Total Carbohydrates 5.4g

Dietary Fiber 1.4g

Sugars 1.1g

Protein 62g

Ingredients

- 4 Chicken Thighs
- 2 Garlic cloves
- 1 Lemon
- 2 tbsp. Butter
- 4 sprigs of Rosemary, fresh
- Pepper & salt to taste

Directions

1. Preheat your oven to 400 F in advance & heat up a cast iron skillet over high heat settings.
2. Generously season the chicken thighs with pepper & salt, preferably on both sides. Carefully place the coated chicken thighs into the hot skillet, preferably skin side down & let them sear for couple of minutes, until nicely brown.
3. Flip the chicken pieces & flavor the thighs by squeezing

half of the lemon. Quarter the leftover lemon halves & throw them into the hot pan.

4. Chop the garlic cloves roughly & add them along with some fresh rosemary to the hot skillet.
5. Place the skillet inside the preheated oven & bake for half an hour.
6. Remove the skillet from the oven & to add flavor, moisture & extra crispiness; feel free to add a small amount of butter over the chicken thighs. Bake for 10 more minutes.
7. Serve with a small amount of sautéed green beans & enjoy.

LAMB MEATBALLS WITH CAULIFLOWER PILAF

Total Preparation & Cooking Time: 30 minutes
Servings: 4

Nutritional Value (Estimated Amount Per Serving)

Calories 531

Calories from Fat 352

Total Fat 39g

Saturated Fat 21g

Trans Fat 0g

Polyunsaturated Fat 2.4g

Monounsaturated Fat 12g

Cholesterol 179mg

Sodium 820mg

Potassium 605mg

Total Carbohydrates 5.9g

Dietary Fiber 2.5g

Sugars 2g

Protein 37g

Ingredients

For Cauliflower Rice:

- ½ pounds cauliflower florets
- Pepper & salt to taste

For Meatballs:

- 1 tsp. fennel seed
- 1 egg, large
- 1 tsp. garlic powder
- 1 pound ground lamb
- 1 tsp. pepper
- 1 tsp. salt
- 1 tsp. paprika

Other Ingredients:

- 4 oz goat cheese

- 1 tbsp. lemon zest, fresh
- 2 tbsp. coconut oil
- 1 garlic clove, minced
- ½ yellow onion, chopped
- A bunch of mint leaves, fresh, chopped roughly

Directions

1. Pulse the cauliflower in a food processor until it looks like rice. Cook the riced-cauliflower in a pan, preferably lightly oiled for 8 minutes, covered. Season with pepper & salt to taste.
2. Combine lamb together with egg & spices in a large-sized bowl. Using your hands; mix them well and make 12 to 15 meatballs from the mixture; set aside.
3. Now, over medium heat settings in a large skillet, heat the coconut oil & cook the onion until translucent, for 5 to 8 minutes.
4. Add in the garlic & let cook for a minute or two, until fragrant.
5. Now, cook all sides of the meatballs in the hot pan. Cook until firm to touch & no longer pink.
6. Evenly divide the cauliflower rice into four portions.
7. Add some of the meatballs to each portion of the cauliflower rice & top with the lemon zest, fresh mint leaves & crumbled goat cheese. Serve & enjoy.

EASY LOBSTER BISQUE

Total Preparation & Cooking Time: 1 hour & 20 minutes
Servings: 4

Nutritional Value (Estimated Amount Per Serving)

Calories 649

Calories from Fat 257

Total Fat 29g

Saturated Fat 15g

Trans Fat 0.7g

Polyunsaturated Fat 2.8g

Monounsaturated Fat 8.5g

Cholesterol 220mg

Sodium 2222mg

Potassium 1053mg

Total Carbohydrates 24g

Dietary Fiber 3.4g

Sugars 10g

Protein 49g

Ingredients

- 1 oz brandy
- 24 oz lobster chunks
- 1 cup heavy cream
- 4 garlic cloves
- 1 tsp. paprika
- ½ red onion
- 1 tsp. xanthan gum
- 2 carrots
- 1 tsp. thyme
- 4 celery stalks
- 1 tsp. peppercorns
- ½ cup tomato paste
- 1 quart seafood broth
- 2 cups white wine
- 1 tbsp. lemon juice, fresh
- 3 bay leaves

- 1 tbsp. olive oil
- Parsley, fresh
- 1 tbsp. salt

Directions

1. Finely chop the garlic, onion, carrots & celery.
2. Over moderate heat settings in a soup pot; heat the olive oil & cook the onion for a minute or two, until fragrant and then add in the garlic & cook until crusty at the bottom & the pan looks slightly blackened. Using the white wine; deglaze the pot & then add in the carrot and celery.
3. Pour in the broth together with tomato paste and brandy; give everything a good stir until well incorporated. Add in the spices & let the soup to simmer for one hour.
4. Once the spices have let out their flavors & the soup has cooked through; remove the bay leaves & discard.
5. Add in the cream & bring it to a simmer again and then add a bit of xanthan gum; continue to stir the soup until thickened.
6. Before adding the lobster chunks; blend the soup and then add in the lobster. Transfer the soup in a large blender & blend on high settings until creamy.
7. Cut the lobster into chunks & sauté in some olive oil or butter in a large saucepan, if uncooked.
8. Transfer the bisque into a large-sized bowl & add in the lobster chunks; give everything a good stir until well combined.
9. Dress the bisque with green onion, lemon juice, parsley or chives. Serve & enjoy.

LOW CARB GNOCCHI

Total Preparation & Cooking Time: 40 minutes
Servings: 2

Nutritional Value (Estimated Amount Per Serving)

Calories 85

Calories from Fat 61

Total Fat 6.8g

Saturated Fat 2.4g

Trans Fat 0g

Polyunsaturated Fat 1.1g

Monounsaturated Fat 3g

Cholesterol 277mg

Sodium 1175mg

Potassium 37mg

Total Carbohydrates 1.5g

Dietary Fiber 0.1g

Sugars 0.2g

Protein 4.2g

Ingredients

- 3 egg yolks
- ½ tsp. garlic powder
- 2 cups mozzarella, shredded, part skim, low moisture
- 1 tsp. salt

Directions

1. Melt the mozzarella with any seasonings in a toaster oven or microwave for 10 minutes, stirring every now and then. Separate the egg yolks from whites & beat them until evenly combined. Pour half of the egg yolks and using two silicone spatulas mix them into the melted mozzarella; combine well.
2. When done, separate it into ¼; rolling each ¼ into a long & thin strip on a piece of parchment paper. Put approximately 1" pieces in each strip until you have a lot of cheese gnocchi. Gently pressing the fork on them.

3. Bring a large pot of water to a boil over moderate heat settings & drop the gnocchi in. Boil until starts floating & then drain. Now, fry the gnocchi on an oiled pan, on both sides. Serve them with some roasted Brussels sprouts & vodka sauce.

CONCLUSION

The ketogenic diet has been proven to be highly beneficial for our bodies and to even control and prevent some serious diseases. The ketogenic diet is based on taking advantage of your body's natural fat burning processes to shed those pounds in no time. Start the diet today and feel the difference within weeks.

62075050R00062

Made in the USA
Middletown, DE
18 January 2018